Better Lives

FOR DISABLED WOMEN

JO CAMPLING
Lecturer in Social Policy, Hillcroft College

Dedication

For my mother who became disabled at the age of three.

Acknowledgements

In writing this book I am indebted to many people especially the disabled women who helped me so generously. I would like to thank Elsa Beckett, Toni Belfield, Angela Blenkinsop, Pamela Boal, Sue Bregman, Rosemary Brotherwood, Heather Connell, John Curtis, Davinia D'Arcy de Nayth, Liz Fanshawe, Mary Greaves, Joanna Johnson, Sally Hale, Ann Hamilton, David Jordan, Philippa Lane, Sarah Lomas, Anne MacFarlane, Dorothy Mandelstam, Jean Nicklin, Don Oswald, Maisie Slack, Bill Stewart, Dana Wilson, George Wilson and Bernice Wood — and Margaret Eades, who did the typing.

Jo Campling

Jo Campling is Lecturer in Social Policy, Hillcroft College and specialises in writing and research on disability.

Published in Great Britain by Virago Limited 1979
5 Wardour Street, London W1V 3HE

Copyright © Jo Campling

ISBN 0 86068 050 9

This book is sold subject to the condition that it shall not, by way of trade or otherwise, be lent, re-sold, hired out or otherwise circulated without the publisher's prior consent in any form of binding or cover other than that in which it is published without a similar condition including this condition being imposed on the subsequent purchaser. This book is published at a net price and is supplied subject to the Publishers Association Standard Conditions of Sale registered under the Restrictive Trades Practices Act, 1956.

Printed and bound by Unwin Brothers Limited,
The Gresham Press, Old Woking, Surrey.

Contents

	Preface	1
	Author's Note	2
	Glossary	3
1	Relationships	5
2	Sexuality and Self-Image	9
3	Menstruation and Menopause	13
4	Contraception	15
5	Pregnancy and Motherhood	17
6	Incontinence	21
7	Clothing	24
8	Women at Home	28
9	Education and Employment	33
10	Benefits	38
11	Where to Get Advice and Help	42
	Further Reading	44

VIRAGO
is a feminist publishing company

'It is only when women start to organize in large numbers that we become a political force, and begin to move towards the possibility of a truly democratic society in which every human being can be brave, responsible, thinking and diligent in the struggle to live at once freely and unselfishly'

SHEILA ROWBOTHAM
Women, Resistance and Revolution

VIRAGO
Advisory Group

Andrea Adam
Carol Adams
Sally Alexander
Anita Bennett
Liz Calder
Bea Campbell
Angela Carter
Mary Chamberlain
Deirdre Clark
Anna Coote
Jane Cousins
Anna Davin
Rosalind Delmar
Zoe Fairbairns
Carolyn Faulder
Germaine Greer
Jane Gregory

Christine Jackson
Suzanne Lowry
Jean McCrindle
Nancy Meiselas (*USA*)
Mandy Merck
Cathy Porter
Elaine Showalter (*USA*)
Spare Rib Collective
Mary Stott
Anne Summers (*Australia*)
Rosalie Swedlin
Michelene Wandor
Alison Weir
Elizabeth Wilson
Women and Education
Barbara Wynn

Preface

I was just an ordinary little girl with fair curly hair wearing pretty dresses made by my mother until suddenly, one day in November when I was three-and-a-half years old I ceased being a little girl and became a 'polio'. Just a few hours and I was 'neutered' — a sexless little creature.

My hair was cut like a boy's (in those days boys didn't have long hair and girls didn't have short hair). I wore boy's jerseys over a nightdress until I was about eight years old. But I wasn't a little boy. One eminent consultant greeted me in those early days with, 'Now, my little man and how are you today?' To which I answered scornfully, 'Mary is a girl's name.' This little incident illustrates what I am sure a great many disabled girls and women feel — they are deprived of their femininity, and in consequence their role as a woman, because of their disability.

It is because of this that a great many disabled women will welcome this book, not only because at last some one has recognised that they face specific problems, not just because they are disabled, but because they are disabled *women*. Jo Campling has not only discussed all aspects of these special problems with imagination and sensitivity, but in addition she suggests practical solutions and provides names and addresses of organisations which may be able to give additional help.

I am sure this book will prove invaluable to many disabled women and to their relatives and friends.

Mary Greaves, 1979.

Mary Greaves, BSc (Econ), M.A., M.B.E., received the Harding Award in 1973 for her work for the improvement of the disabled in society. She is the author of 'Work and Disability'.

Author's note

The original plan of action for the United Nations Decade for Women, 1975-1985, included the intention to study measures which would help disabled women lead more fulfilling lives. The measure was dropped because it is not yet generally recognised that many of the problems of handicapped women stem from, or are an extension of, discrimination against *all* women, and that to be female and disabled in our society is a double drawback. Yet in Great Britain alone there are more than twice as many handicapped women as men. This is partly due to the fact that women live longer than men and many of their disabilities are connected with ageing, but also that some disabilities affect women more often than men. For example over 60 per cent of people suffering from multiple sclerosis which affects the younger age group, are women. Women are also more affected, professionally and personally, as the careers of those who are disabled.

It is impossible to generalise about disabled women, and amongst those so defined there is great diversity. The handicap may be hidden or obvious, a common or rare condition, disabling in only one area of activity or affecting a whole way of life. It may be a static condition like polio or a progressive one, like multiple sclerosis. There may be physiological abnormality or loss, through surgery or an accident, as in most spinal cord injuries. Or it may be a chronic condition like rheumatoid arthritis which alters or interrupts normal physiological processes. Or it may be a congenital defect like spina bifida, which inhibits these same processes. Whatever the cause, manifestation and degree of the disability, they all involve a limitation of ordinary activity, which may mean an incapacity for self-care and management and perhaps an inability to walk, wash and dress, for example. It will also mean a significant change in the way a woman sees herself and is seen by others.

I wrote this book to focus attention on aspects of disability rarely discussed. I have attempted to bring together a discussion of the considerable social and psychological difficulties faced by adult disabled women who live at home, the practical problems they face, and how to cope with them.

SIMPLE DEFINITIONS OF COMMON DISABILITIES

Cerebral Palsy. Cerebral palsy is a medical term given to a group of neurological conditions, that is, conditions to do with the nervous system. They all involve a disorder of motor control to varying degrees, the result of injury or disease of the brain, before, during or sometimes after, birth. A person with cerebral palsy is known as spastic. There is no cure for cerebral palsy because brain damage is normally irreversible.

Multiple Sclerosis (MS). Progressive disease of unknown origin which affects the central nervous system, causing varying degrees of paralysis, impaired vision, slurred speech and bladder and bowel weakness. It is one of the most common causes of crippling in adults. More women are affected than men, in the proportion of three to two. A characteristic of the disease, despite its progressive nature, is periods of remission of the symptoms.

Muscular Dystrophy. There are several kinds of muscular dystrophy. All are progressive, wasting diseases of the voluntary muscles. The results are increasing weakness and loss of muscle bulk which causes difficulty in walking and in the use of arms.

Poliomyelitis (Polio). This is an acute infection of the central nervous system, often resulting in paralysis. If the disease does not respond to treatment, one or all of the affected limbs remain paralysed. Some people suffer complete paralysis and have to rely on breathing apparatus to keep them alive. In Britain polio is not the killer disease it once was.

Rheumatoid Arthritis. Progressive disease of unknown origin which affects multiple joints of the body causing swelling, severe pain, destruction of the joint and deformity. More women than men have rheumatoid arthritis of the extremities but more men than women have the spinal form.

Spina Bifida. Congenital defect resulting from incomplete formation of the spinal column resulting in injury to the cord. The consequences of the malformation are paralysis of the legs and absence or weakness of control of bladder and bowels. Three-quarters of those with spina bifida also develop hydrocephalus, an excess of fluid in the brain. This condition also occurs independently. Since 1958 it has been possible to treat hydrocephalus.

Spinal Cord Injury. The spinal cord, which lies inside the protective bony spine, is a continuation of the nerve cells and bundles of the brain, and carries its messages. Therefore the place of injury to the spinal cord is the determining factor in the degree of physical disability. The higher the injury, the worse the effects. A broken neck or fracture at the top of the spine causes paralysis of arms and legs. If the injury is at waist level or lower, the upper part of the body will not be paralysed. Paralysis of both arms and legs is quadriplegia. Paralysis of both legs is called paraplegia.

Stroke. This is the result of damage to part of the brain caused by an interruption to its blood supply. Strokes are so called because they usually occur rapidly. It is as if the illness suddenly 'strikes'. There are several other names used such as apoplexy, shock, spasm, seizure, cerebral thrombosis, cerebral haemorrhage or cerebro-vascular accident. Strokes can result in paralysis of one side of the body (hemiplegia) or slight loss of strength in one arm or leg (hemiparesis). The degree of recovery varies from person to person, depending on the severity of the stroke. Some people get better completely, whilst some patients do not survive the first few days.

1 Relationships

It may be difficult or impossible for a handicapped woman to fulfil the recognised female roles. Yet society will expect her to behave in certain approved or stereotyped ways as a disabled person and as a woman. Both involve a socially defined position and status which inspires a mixture of discrimination, condescension and consideration. And irrespective of her behaviour or condition, she will attract certain kinds of attention by virtue of the fact that she is disabled and a woman. It is rare to find that she is treated as an ordinary member of the community without this sort of separation occurring. For some women, this may not be unwelcome. It may be easier to accept dependency, to ask for help to carry a wheelchair downstairs or put it into a car, to be lifted and given physical help. For others, particularly where disability occurs in later life, it requires a drastic redefinition of life-style and status in their private and public life, to which adjustment is painful and difficult.

Within the family, the wife and mother tends to be the person who bears the major emotional and supportive responsibility for all its members. It may not be possible for the disabled woman to continue this role. Disability affects not just the victim but the whole family. The impact of one member of the family being disabled means alterations in the whole family structure and relationships. A man may tend to feel more threatened by financial dependency through the loss of his role as a breadwinner, but a woman is likely to be more anxious about losing her supportive role in the family. The question of dependency is crucial, as every disabled person, male or female, has to face it. The relationship between childhood dependency and disabled dependency can be emphasised by some aids and equipment, for example the similarities between a wheelchair and a pram. In one study a woman was distressed because her daughter said that her mother's incontinence pads looked like nappies. A woman may find that the family is so anxious about her disability that they become over-protective and family reaction may set the seal on how she sees herself. This may be particularly true of disabled women who live with their parents. Often the price of family harmony seems to be an acceptance of a dependent or subordinate role by the disabled woman. However, social relationships are flexible, and roles can be re-negotiated if the family are aware of this. Women living alone face different problems of dependency, isolation and change of role.

Sometimes a disabled woman, single or married, living alone or with others, will feel forced by family, friends and even professionals into an acceptance of an inferior role or status, and thus feel stigmatised and devalued. The question of stigma is important. Throughout history the physically handicapped, with other groups like the mentally ill and the poor, have been stigmatised as inferior and have been seen as helpless dependants. Goffman defined the term stigma in this context as 'an individual who might have been received easily in ordinary social intercourse, but possesses a trait that can obtrude itself upon the attention and turn those of us whom she meets away from her, breaking the claim that her other attributes have on us.' In this way the able-bodied exercise discrimination which reduces the quality of life of the disabled. The woman will feel stigmatised by the reactions and sanctions of family, friends colleagues and professionals, so that it becomes a major problem, not only to cope with the physical effects of disability, but with the social and psychological consequences. It is these which produce a negative self-image.

One of the major problems of the disabled woman is coming to terms with a spoiled body image, because this is the visible sign of her disability and a focus of stigma. Assessment of appearance is the starting point in interaction with other people. In our society there is an ideal of desirable physical appearance. Outward appearance is often particularly important to women. A physically handicapped woman may have difficulty with her self-care and personal toilet which causes distress. Additionally, the presence of a wheelchair, callipers or stick puts her into the category of handicapped and other people will react accordingly. Several types of behaviour are adopted to contend with the reactions of others to disability. One is an attempt to hide the visible signs of impairment, known as 'passing'. Another is 'normalisation' in which she pretends that things are not as hard as they appear. In other words she is challenging the commonly held expectations about the handicapped and is saying 'my disability is not my main attribute or my total identity'. The social significance of the disability is being rejected rather than the disability itself. This strategy does not always work, if for example, she is asked to dance or has to seek help in some revealing way. 'Withdrawal' or 'dissociation' from social interaction is another method of coping and is used to protect against embarrassment or rejection. However, it is dangerous, as too often it means social isolation. The woman becomes separated from former relationships and activities. Sometimes the withdrawal is by friends and acquaintances rather than by the disabled woman herself. It has often been noted how friendship circles change after disability. Many able-bodied people are unable to cope with

physical disability in their friends or members of their family.
　　None of these strategies for coping are peculiar to the disabled woman. Able-bodied people also use them in every day life to sustain their own self-images. The difference is that they are used only for short periods when their identity is under stress or threat. For the disabled woman these methods of coping may become a way of life which confirm her negative self-image and prevent her rehabilitation.

MARRIAGE

Disability in a woman affects the family in many ways. No aspect of family life is immune. Social aspects can change quickly as friendships are altered or lost. The economic life of the family may be changed, especially where the wife is also a breadwinner or the husband has to neglect his work in order to look after her. The nature of family interactions will not be the same, and the family may no longer have the social and psychological cohesion it had. Disability may create role ambiguity and role reversal, especially where the woman has been the mainstay and support of the family as wife and mother. It has often been said that it is easier for a disabled woman to adopt a dependent role than a disabled man, that this is more acceptable within the female sex-role stereotype. This is not always so, and a woman who has spent all her life in the role of carer will find it difficult to come to terms with the change. In any case the dynamics of marriage and family living involve a complex range of delicate, emotional nuances which even challenge the adjustment process of the non-disabled. Marital and family adjustment is difficult enough with the able-bodied. When a disability is added, the difficulties imposed by the handicap may distort the situation.
　　Certainly the difficulties of couples vary according to whether one or both partners are disabled, whether disability came before or after the marriage, whether the marriage was a stable one before disability, the age at which disability developed, the severity of the handicap and whether or not there are children. Most partnerships between people disabled at the time of marriage appear to have a higher chance of stability than the 50 per cent chance which able-bodied people possess. But when disability occurs in one partner after marriage, there is a much higher chance of break-up. The onset of disability in a marriage is a crisis. The better adjusted two people are in their total relationship before the crisis, the better able they are to readjust their relationship afterwards. Marital and personal

difficulties which have been concealed or ignored in the past may become obvious or heightened. Even where there is no question of divorce both the disabled partner and the non-disabled admit a deterioration in marital satisfaction. The strongest of marriages will come under strain. It may not be easy for the husband to accept the physical changes in his wife, or for her to accept her own disability and change of role in the partnership. Sexual difficulty or deprivation can adversely affect the whole structure of the marriage. The question of roles is crucial. It is not easy for the disabled woman to be both patient and sexual partner in a relationship which now involves both, or for her husband to fulfil the role of nurse and lover. On her side, diminished self-esteem, fear of the loss of the husband's love and support, and on both sides feelings of deprivation and frustration may follow the realisation that the old roles can no longer be enacted. The problems which follow are often more severe because they are often unexpressed. For the disabled wife they may be exacerbated because of attitudes to traditional female roles, the misinformation about women's sexuality in general and ignorance about disabled people's sexual abilities in particular.

2 Sexuality and self-image

The psychological effect of physical disablement on a person's self-image can be devastating, whether male or female. But the female condition, idealised by many cultures as nurturing, responsive and attractive to men, carries added pressures for the disabled woman. Her ability to give sexual pleasure, to be, as well as to look, sexually inviting is a basic part of her conditioning from childhood. Additionally, for many people a woman's role and her femininity still often depends on her ability to be a wife and mother. Acceptance of disability, learning to see oneself as a sexual being and as a person worth relating to, are all important to self-esteem. Many disabled women have poor self-images, partly because of the attitudes of others towards them. One woman has described how, as an adolescent, her boyfriend would take her out in a wheelchair. Everyone assumed that she must be his relative, because they could not accept her as a typical girl able to attract a boy friend.

In recent years Masters and Johnson, *The Hite Report* and more especially the women's movement have raised questions about female sexuality. Theories about women's role, passivity, maternal needs and instincts and the nature of the female orgasm have all been challenged. Sexuality is not just the act of intercourse, it involves the whole business of relating to another human being and a wide range of communication and activity. The difficulties experienced by most women in determining their own sexuality are intensified if that woman is disabled. Sexuality springs from a good self-image and enhances one's self-esteem. For disabled women, valuing themselves enough to accept their sexuality can be the first step towards a fuller life. If there is a common denominator of disabled women's sexual problems, it is in the area of self-image. In a society where physical attractiveness in women is valued so highly, especially through the mass media, a negative value is placed on a physical defect and a damaged or distorted self-image results.

Society finds it difficult on the whole, to cope with the idea of a disabled woman having the same emotional needs and desires as other women. Much of the published material on sex for the disabled. does not deal with female sexuality as such, or deals with it in very traditional ways, that is emphasising female passivity and the fact that a woman need not have an orgasm in order to be able to satisfy her partner. Gunnel Enby, a Swedish wife and mother who had polio at sixteen, has noted how people were often surprised that she functioned successfully as a sexual being despite her paralysis and wheelchair. She attributed this perception of her as sexually impotent to lack of knowledge and lack of contact with disabled people. Indeed, contrary to the myths, there is now accumulating clinical and research data to suggest that sexual adjustment is at the core of the psychological rehabilitation process.

Sexuality exists for everyone, not to be dismissed because of crutches, wheelchairs, scars or spasms. As Anna Freud said, 'Sex is something we do. Sexuality is something we are.' The sexual needs of disabled women have been ignored for too long. It is true that disability may inhibit a satisfactory sex life for a woman by making normal intercourse difficult or impossible, by restricting her choice of contraception and making pregnancy and child-rearing problematic. But the need to love and be loved is important for everyone — it is not the prerogative of the able-bodied. There are many ways of expressing love and sexuality with or without full intercourse and orgasm. A woman may need to learn and practise new ways of loving and caring which can provide a sense of well-being and intimacy as fulfilling as for an able-bodied woman, though not necessarily in the same ways.

SEXUAL ACTIVITY

The disabled woman may have special problems affecting the expression of her sexuality. For some women who are handicapped a nearly normal and satisfactory sex life is possible. For others, altered forms of sexual activity may be necessary depending on the degree to which she can feel and move, how much pain she has, whether she has spasms, urinary and bowel difficulties. For all, a major consideration involves the need for greater communication in order that the disabled woman can let her partner know how to both help and please her. Realistically, the partners must assess the nature and extent of the disability and its limitations on what they can and cannot do sexually. One way of doing this is through personal experimentation, although doctors and counsellors can also help. Once the limitations are understood a pattern of sex within these limits can be worked out. Traditional genital intercourse with only some variations in positioning is possible for many. For others sexual activity may have to be limited to non-coital techniques such as touching, kissing, petting, or oral genital stimulation.

In our society an order of sexual activity is still generally recognised as passing from kissing to caressing to penile penetration of the vagina. This is not necessarily the most satisfying sexually from the woman's point of view, and intercourse and good sexual relations are not necessarily synonymous. It is important to realise that oral and manual expressions of sex are neither perverted nor unused by able-bodied people. Research has shown that exceptionally few sexual acts are dangerous or hazardous to health. The woman who is disabled should engage in any sexual activity which is physiologically possible, pleasurable and acceptable to her and her partner. The only criteria for concern should be what the two people prefer within their own limitations.

For sexual activity it is essential to be able to find a comfortable position. The 'missionary' position with the woman on her back and the man on top of her may not be possible. Or it may be easier to put pillows beneath the knees and buttocks. For some, lying on the side either facing her partner or with her back to him is more comfortable. For others, lying on the stomach with the man on top may be best. Where spasms are a problem it is better to take a position where these are less likely to occur, for example, lying face down. For still others, a standing or kneeling position, resting against a chair could be comfortable. Where lubrication is a problem a jelly such as K-Y should be used (rather than vaseline which can cause vaginal infection). One of the most embarrassing complications for disabled women is urinary or bowel incontinence. For the woman with a catheter (a tube which is passed into the bladder to draw off urine) which cannot be safely removed during intercourse, the tube can be taped to the stomach or loin with elastoplast to keep it out of the way. If it can be kept in, this is obviously easier and does avoid the risk of infection. It is quite safe to leave an ileostomy bag where it is quite firmly in place. It should be emptied before intercourse to avoid accidents and can then be taped to the stomach in the same way.

Where genital sex is not possible, erotic touching or oral sex may be the most pleasurable activity. This is using the mouth or the tongue. Where no feeling exists in the sexual organs, it is often found that other parts of the body increase in sexual feeling. In these circumstances, extreme pleasure can be obtained by stroking and caressing the breasts, neck or other parts of the body. It is important for a woman to understand her own body and to know which areas are still sensitive to sexual arousal when stimulated. Women can still experience orgasm even when a significant part of their bodies may be without sensation or motion. Orgasm can happen through fantasy, breast stimulation or other means. Women who are never orgasmic or rarely experience orgasm may find sexual satisfaction in other ways. It may be emotional or spiritual rather than physical. The sexual act does not exist in isolation but as one element in the total activity of a couple. For some women the psychological aspects of a relationship create sufficient satisfaction. There is a need for great sensitivity, understanding and compensatory activity between two people who love each other but are limited in the pleasure they can share in the physical sense. A deep and satisfying relationship can exist even when unimpeded sexual activity is not possible. As one woman said, 'Sex may end in the penis, but it starts in the mind'.

The need to be more open and experimental can lead couples to discover a range of touching, positions and pleasures which able-bodied couples might never discover. Disability can have the effect of forcing a couple to be completely honest with themselves and with each other, leading to that 'exchange of mutual vulnerabilities' which Masters and Johnson saw as central in loving relationships.

The Committee on Sexual Problems of the Disabled, known as SPOD publishes a series of excellent leaflets and provides an advisory and counselling service (see p. 42). The Family Planning Association will also advise and has suitable publications (see p. 43).

For disabled women who are lesbian there are the added problems of the attitude of society and the difficulty of finding a partner. Few disabled women feel that they can let family and friends know that they relate sexually to women, so their isolation is intensified. For this reason *Gemma,* a group for disabled and non-disabled homosexual women was formed in 1976. It is not a counselling service nor a gay dating agency but simply a group of friends with some understanding, through their own experiences, of the difficulties facing disabled lesbian women. They can be contacted at BM Box 5700, London W1C1V 6XX. Another organisation helping disabled gay men and women is Gaycare which can be contacted at 2a Thirlmere Road, Streatham, London SW16.

Many women find masturbation a comforting and pleasurable experience. Masturbation is a totally harmless activity, a means of self exploration which can help to show a woman what her body can feel and express and may help her to communicate to others what gives her pleasure. It is not necessarily genital and can involve other parts of the body. Masturbation may be difficult or painful for women with arthritis or high spinal cord injuries. However, where it is possible and does not conflict with personal feelings or beliefs, it can enlarge sexual experience for disabled women.

3 Menstruation and menopause

For disabled women, periods do present extra problems. Generally speaking, the menstrual cycle is unaffected by disability. An exception is spinal cord injury where periods often stop for several months, but later resume normally. Evidence suggests that girls who are born with a disability menstruate earlier than able-bodied girls. A case has been reported of a spina bifida girl starting her periods at six years old. This can present problems, since sex education rarely begins until at least eleven years old. On the other hand a woman who has grown up with a disability may even welcome menstruation. As one woman said, 'At last my body has done something right, something every female body is supposed to do'.

Nevertheless the problems are considerable, particularly for the wheelchair bound or where there is restricted use of the hands. Tampons may provide better protection than sanitary towels, which can easily slip out of place. They are also less likely to cause smell. It may be necessary to slide to the edge of the wheelchair in order to insert a tampon, or to insert it from the rear whilst seated on the toilet. For some disabilities insertion on the back, side or in a reclining position will be easier.

If feeling has been impaired in the pelvic area, menstrual pains may be mild or non-existent. Where periods are a real problem because of inability to change sanitary towels, insert a tampon, or wash, or where pre-menstrual congestion, period pains or excessive bleeding are severe, suppression of the periods may be considered by the doctor. Often the use of one of the combined contraceptive pills is the most satisfactory solution. Continuous hormone therapy or a radium menopause have problems of adverse side-effects, so in some cases a hysterectomy may be the treatment of choice.

Between forty-five and fifty-five the menopause takes place. Menstrual periods stop and pregnancy is no longer a possibility. Often the menopause is accompanied by uncomfortable physical symptoms due to hormonal changes, such as depression, vaginal dryness and hot flushes. There is no evidence of a difference in these symptoms between disabled and able-bodied women.

Hormone replacement therapy (HRT) (see FPA, p 43) can give relief from some of the more troublesome symptoms of the menopause. However currently this form of treatment is the subject of debate because of significant side-effects. Dosage has to be carefully measured and monitored on an individual basis, as women vary in their oestrogen levels. There is some evidence which links HRT with breast and uterine cancer. Each woman and her doctor must weigh the risks against the benefits in order to decide if it is acceptable.

4 Contraception

Fertility is rarely affected by a disability, so suitable methods of contraception need to be investigated. If, on the other hand, a disabled woman is sure that she will never want children for any reason, she may consider voluntary sterilisation, which involves surgical cutting and tying of the Fallopian tubes. This operation is generally considered to be irreversible, but does not alter a woman's periods, sexual drive or responsiveness. In some cases the male partner may choose to have a vasectomy, a simple operation to cut and tie the sperm duct. (This operation is sometimes reversible).

Some disabled women may choose the rhythm method, that is, abstaining from intercourse during the fertile period. There are no health risks, but there is a much higher chance of pregnancy than with most other methods. Also, record-keeping and temperature-taking can be difficult for a woman with limited manual dexterity. Or the man may use the sheath, alone or in conjunction with pessaries (jellies, creams or tablets placed in the vagina) and chemical agents, but these will be impractical if the woman does not have the full use of her hands and arms. Similarly the diaphragm or cap may be difficult to insert for a woman with restricted use of her hands, unless she relies on her partner. It does take practice to feel comfortable using this method and if pelvic muscles are weak the diaphragm may slip. On the other hand it can be inserted in advance and if menstruation is a concern during intercourse, it can be used to contain the flow. Introduction of an intra-uterine device (IUD), the coil, a plastic or metal object inserted by the doctor into the uterus, may be difficult where there is pain or restricted movement of the hips. IUDs can bring on heavier periods, causing problems in coping with personal hygiene. There is an increased risk of pelvic inflammatory disease and a woman who lacks feeling in her pelvic area might not notice its warning signs. However it is fair to say that many women experience no side effects or discomfort with the device.

For some disabled women, an oral contraceptive or pill may be the method of choice for family planning, although care is needed in selecting a pill with a hormonal content best suited to the particular individual. The advantages are that it requires no measures in conjunction with intercourse and is extremely safe as a method of birth control. However, the use of the pill has been statistically shown to entail a small but increased risk of thrombosis (blood clots). Paralysis can result in circulatory problems, and some disabled women will not feel the warning signs such as severe leg, arm or abdominal pains. A few women feel depressed, have headaches, gain weight whilst on the pill, which may be extra problems to someone trying to cope with disability. On the other side, an advantage can be the reduction in menstrual flow, a boon to the woman in a wheelchair. There is no research on the side-effects of oral contraceptives for disabled women, although this is clearly needed. Another alternative is the mini-pill, which is often effective for women who experience the oestrogen-related side-effects of the pill, but it is not known if there is a greater risk of blood clots with these progesterone-only pills. Irregular periods and spotting can happen with this method but periods may stop altogether, which is convenient if menstruation is a problem.

An answer for some disabled women may be depo-provera (D-P), a progesterone-only injection given every three months, and with a pregnancy risk the same as the pill. However, it is not available everywhere and to date there is no product licence for its long-term use and it is used mainly as a short-term method of contraception. An association has been found between D-P and cervical cancer, and there is a possibility of infertility especially if it is taken for some time. The return to fertility may also take longer than with oral contraceptives, so doctors may be particularly reluctant to give it to women who want to be pregant at a later date.

Whatever choice of contraceptive is made it is essential that careful advice is taken and that the prescribing doctor is fully aware of the individual's medical history. The Family Planning Association have a number of useful leaflets and publications and a full list can be obtained from them. They also offer a comprehensive information and advice service (see p. 43).

5 Pregnancy and motherhood

There are many misunderstandings and taboos surrounding motherhood and disability, but a major issue for many disabled women is the right to have children. Few disabilities are hereditary. For example, there is no reason why a woman disabled as the result of polio should not have children. Women who are orthopaedically handicapped do not usually have more difficult pregnancies or deliveries than other women. For some women, for example the rheumatoid patient, pregnancy may produce a sense of well-being and a remission of symptoms, although delivery may be followed by their exacerbation. Women with multiple sclerosis (MS) may have children but this is not always recommended because there is some evidence to suggest that MS symptoms may become aggravated with pregnancy. A study in Sweden in 1963 by Guttman has shown that paraplegics have given birth without complication to healthy children. Where there is no hereditary disability a handicapped woman is no more likely to have an abnormal child than an able-bodied woman. Even if a woman becomes disabled during pregnancy, it is unlikely that the baby will suffer harm although it may arrive rather early.

However, it is essential to have genetic counselling where there is any chance at all that disability can be inherited, for example women who have dystrophies of genetic origin. In most cases the GP will be able to put the woman's mind at rest. If specialist advice is required she should be referred to the nearest Genetic Advisory Centre by her GP. She may have to be persistent in her enquiries. Often a genetic counsellor is able to calculate the risk of transmitted disability accurately on family history alone, or sometimes in conjunction with simple tests on both partners. Further information can be obtained from a booklet published by the Department of Health and Social Security (DHSS) called *Human Genetics*

It is important that disabled women have their babies in hospital. Labour does not often present any complications but premature births do occur more often. Sometimes the mother is unable to bear down, as in the case of a woman with cerebral palsy, or there may be difficulty in expulsion due to spasms or cramps in the muscles of the pelvic area and a Caesarian may be necessary. Any woman who has severe restriction of movement and pain in the hips, knees or spine, or where a normal labour is inadvisable, may have delivery by Caesarian section. Any physical change after the birth which the woman experiences should be reported to her doctor, as there can be various post-natal problems. For example, childbirth inevitably imposes a strain on the pelvic muscles, but many disabled women cannot do the post-natal exercises and this may lead to bladder and bowel incontinence.

Whilst no one has the right to prevent a disabled woman having children, she should be aware of the implications and responsibilities when she may be physically unable to cope with them. Indeed doctors will often discourage a woman on the grounds that the child may suffer and that the woman would not be able to cope with emergencies. A physical handicap is not necessarily a handicap to being a parent. Being a parent involves not only the practical care of the child, but also giving it emotional security and love. On the other hand a disabled mother may run into difficulties if she has not taken into consideration her own limitations and the extent of the help she is able to rely on from her partner, family, friends and the social services.

Preparation during pregnancy is important. The question of alterations and aids to help with the day-to-day care of the baby need to be investigated. Some of these may well be provided by the local authority and usually the Health Visitor, who always visits after the birth of a baby, can put the mother into contact with the relevant person in Social Services (which can be found in the telephone book under your area in London, or under 'Social Services' outside London). The Health Visitor is a vital contact for all aspects of baby care. She will advise about feeding. For instance a mother on permanent medication must ensure that none of her drugs, if transmitted to the baby in her milk, will be harmful. A healthy wheelchair mother may have a tendency to over-produce milk because of her sedentary existence instead of the more usual problem of an inadequate supply in an over-tired, able-bodied mother. There are practical advantages to breast feeding for the disabled mother. The milk is prepared without the need for sterilisation and at the right temperature. The mother is given a close physical relationship with the baby, even if she has only one or no arms and cannot cuddle him in the usual sense. Where bottle feeding is the choice there is equipment to suit particular disabilities. For example, bottle holders are not manufactured but they can be made from a light metal strip or heavy plastic. They are particularly useful for a 'foot' (someone who can't use her hands at all) mother or one with only a poor grip in the hands.

It is important for the disabled woman that her partner shares the task of caring for the baby. Much of the baby's normal routine, such as bathing, may be difficult for a physically handicapped woman to manage on her own. Problems of tiredness, both during pregnancy and after, common to most mothers, may be even more severe for the woman whose physical resources are already stretched to the limit. Even if she has not needed help before, she may need a home help to assist with the housework while she cares for the baby. The GP or the Health Visitor will advise about this service. All mothers need to be organised, but the disabled mother even more so. She needs to plan carefully and be realistic about her degree of independence. It is wise to economise on energy by handing over difficult tasks where this is possible. Many young babies sleep a lot so this time can be used for rest periods. Equipment should be arranged so that it is near at hand and easily accessible. A trolley is useful to keep all the baby things together. The Disabled Living Foundation (DLF) has published *Early Years* (see p. 43) which gives excellent practical advice on all aspects of baby and child care for the disabled mother. The National Fund for Research into Crippling Diseases also publishes a booklet in their series 'Equipment for the Disabled' called *Disabled Mother* (see p. 43) which has helpful suggestions on how to plan the nursery, the bathroom and so on to enable the mother to cope.

Children adapt to situations that are presented to them and all children accept disability more easily than adults. Mothers who become handicapped after having a family will find that the handicap is soon accepted by their children. And mothers who are already handicapped will find the situation even easier. Children have a natural curiosity but once this has been satisfied, they rarely ask questions. The child of a disabled mother will probably not think her mother any different from her friend's mother. I never noticed that my mother was disabled, and was always surprised when anyone asked why she had funny legs and wore boots.

Safety of her children does not seem to present insoluble problems for the disabled mother. In theory it could be very hazardous for these children, but they seem to develop an instinctive reaction when they know that they have to save themselves. This does not mean that practical safety precautions can be neglected, but children of disabled mothers do not seem to have a higher rate of accidents than other children. As far as discipline is concerned, the disabled mother cannot depend on physical strength and speed but must rely on persuasion.

Activities with young children are often strenuous and demanding, and the handicapped mother may find some beyond her capabilities. In the Amelia Harris survey (see p. 44) it was discovered that this leads to problems of an emotional nature. Playing with children and sharing their leisure is a psychological rather than a physical need on the part of both mother and child, which, because of lack of mobility disabled women may not be able to share outside the home in the same way as other mothers. There are compensations. A disabled woman can give her baby much more attention than the woman who is always busy working or going to the shops. As she is confined to the house she can devote herself more to her child. She is an ideal position to read to her and the child may acquire a wide vocabulary. Barbara Shellard, a disabled mother herself, tells how her son spoke in sentences at thirteen months old and she is sure that this is because she read to him from the age of five months. Loneliness can be a problem for any mother with young children, but more especially for the disabled woman who cannot simply walk down to the shops or the park with her pram. Barbara Shellard advises any prospective mother to try to build up a circle of friends with babies, especially from her own ante-natal classes or maternity hospital. Their children will be the same ages as her own and these mothers could well be a source of support and companionship in the future.

USEFUL PUBLICATIONS

Wendy Greengross, *Entitled to Love,* Malaby Press in association with National Fund for Research into Crippling Diseases 1976.
Towards Intimacy, The Task Force on Concerns of Physically Disabled Women. Family planning and sexuality concerns of physically disabled women. Available from Human Sciences Press, 3 Henrietta Street, London WC2E 8LU, 1978.
Gunnel Enby, *Let There Be Love,* Translated from the Swedish by Irene D. Morris, Taplinger Publishing Company, New York 1975.
I. Nordqvist, *Life Together,* Swedish Central Committee for Rehabilitation (SVRC) 1972.
K. Heslinga *et al, Not Made of Stone ; the sexual problems of handicapped people,* Staflens Scientific Publishing Co. 1974.
Bill Stewart, *Sex and Spina Bifida,* The Association for Spina Bifida and Hydrocephalus, written mainly for young people and their parents. 1978.

6 Incontinence

Incontinence is a taboo subject. The process of the elimination of waste matter from the body is not considered a subject for polite society. From an early age the young child is taught that control of this function is vital in order to gain his parent's approval and that the lack of control is unacceptable and even dirty. The child also learns that this elimination is a private matter and that difficulties or failures are not made public. Girls appear to be particularly fastidious and there is evidence to suggest that they become toilet trained at an earlier age than boys. Women have a keener sense of smell than men, dependent upon the circulatory levels of oestrogen.

Disabled women have more problems where incontinence is concerned than disabled men because of the physiological differences between them. For men there are simple appliances which fit on to, or over, the penis. Urine is collected in a bag strapped to the leg and concealed inside the trouser leg. There are no satisfactory appliances for women to wear. In some cases the doctor may decide that an indwelling catheter (a tube passed into the bladder to draw off urine) is advisable. Usually, however, absorbent pads and protective pants are used in the absence of any comfortable and efficient appliance. Some pants are made of plastic, some of a specially treated nylon fabric (duralite) and there is one type made of hydrophobic (one-way) fabric. There are complaints about the efficiency and discomfort of pants and pads. Their bulk too is unpopular and this may be because of the reminders of nappies and babyhood. Garments which involve depending on others to change the absorptive material induce feelings of humiliation. There is a need for more research on controlling and managing incontinence in women to improve this situation. Doctors will recommend catheters for a severely disabled woman where the effects of sitting on wet padding may be more harmful than the side effects (infection) of catheterisation. There is some risk of infection associated with long-term catheterisation, but incontinence itself may be associated with urinary infection and bed sores.

Pads and pants can be obtained through the District Nurse or local clinic, but the range may be limited. Local chemists stock certain makes, or will order others. In case of difficulty, or if preferred, they can be obtained by mail order. (For a list of stockists and any other information write to the Incontinence Adviser at the

DLF, address p. 43).

Some women find protective pants hot and uncomfortable. For them, Kanga Pants which feel like ordinary pants, may be a solution. They are made of soft, one-way fabric which allows the urine to pass through to be absorbed by a special Kanga pad which is held in a plastic pouch on the outside of the garment. Provided the pad is changed regularly the pants and the body of the wearer remain dry. The pad can be changed without removing the pants and the pants can be washed by hand or machine. Kanga pants are available with Velcro side fastenings for handicapped wearers (see Clothing section) e.g., spina bifida or severe arthritis sufferers. Velcro side fastenings enable the garment to be put on without removing calipers and also give 2 inches of adjustment on each side of the garment enabling a good fit even with severely deformed women. For women with a lesser degree of incontinence there are Kanga Fancy Pants and Bikini pants which are indistinguishable from a normal garment in use and do not require special pads, just a sanitary towel to give the necessary absorbency. Other protective pants have their own special pads, either washable or disposable. An Inco roll, which can be obtained on prescription, can be used to make pads of any desired size and thickness.

If the quantity of urine lost is not great a pad may be sufficient on its own. Ordinary sanitary towels, some of which have self-adhesive tabs for attaching to pants, or a Nikini jock-strap type pant, are useful for slight dribbling. The Cellulose Pad looks like an ordinary sanitary towel, but it contains a substance which gells when wet, and also a deodorant. It will absorb about three times as much fluid as an average pad of similar size. These can be ordered through chemists or may be supplied through clinics. There are also fully disposable pant-and-pad protection of various makes, including the 'Cumfie' which has self-fastening patches, easily used when the woman is confined to a bed or chair. There are also disposable pants made of lightweight non-woven fabric which can be worn over Cumfies for greater security for the less disabled.

There are several types of urinal designed especially for women, including the St Peter's Boat, a pointed dish with a handle which can be slipped easily between the legs. A device of particular use when travelling can be made at home from a flexible plastic funnel with a short length of plastic tubing attached. This can empty into a hot water bottle or another convenient container. Tubings and funnels of different sizes are easily obtainable from hardware shops, large chemists like Boots, where they will usually be found in the wine-making section, or even the aquarian section of pet shops. A new versatile type of urinal, the Feminal, has recently become available. It consists of a moulded plastic section, contoured to fit

the female body, with a short handle in front by means of which it
can be held comfortably and firmly in position. A disposable plastic
bag with an elasticated top fits over the rim and is suspended from it
to collect the urine. It can be used while sitting, standing or lying
down, and it is possible to stand it down quite safely after use
without risk of spilling as the moulded section has straight sides. The
bag can be emptied, disposed of or if necessary, re-used. Feminal is
small and light and could be carried in a handbag.

For women who are incontinent the right choice of clothing
can make the condition more manageable. Modern synthetics which
are easily washed and dried are a boon. Women who wear protective
padding may find a loose fitting tunic or jacket over slacks or skirt
a suitable style. Skirts and nightdresses which open at the back are
more suitable for those confined to chair or bed. For women using a
catheter, a long narrow apron folded up at the bottom to form a
pocket to hold the collecting bag can be tied round the waist under
a fairly long full skirt or caftan. Some may prefer a leg-bag (fastened
on to the leg) under slacks or the Shepheard Sporran, an adjustable
waistbelt which supports a specially designed drainage bag incorporating a drainage outlet.

With both the appliances and clothing, each individual will
need to experiment to see which suits her best. Advice can be
obtained from the DLF.

USEFUL PUBLICATIONS

Dorothy A. Mandelstam, *Incontinence: a guide to the understanding and management of a very common complaint,* for the DLF by Heinemann Health Books 1977.
Peter Lowthian, *Portable Urinals and Related Appliances: a guide to availability and use,* DLF 1975.
Patricia Dobson, *Management of Incontinence in the Home: a survey,* DLF 1974.

7 Clothing

Clothing is a most important part of life for everyone. To some extent individuals are assessed at first sight by their mode of dress. Clothing is often an indication of the wearer's social and economic status. The colour and design of clothes can express the wearer's personality and can be a source of pleasure and satisfaction, in addition to contributing to the maintenance of self-esteem. Unattractive or uncomfortable clothing can spoil the enjoyment of a social occasion. Dressing oneself is essential for independent living. Yet dressing and undressing can be a source of pain and embarrassment to disabled people, of all ages. Unsolved clothing and dressing problems can contribute to a person becoming housebound, or can make it difficult to take a job. They can inhibit normal social life and greatly increase living expenses. Clothing difficulties are therefore a much more important area in the life of disabled people than have previously been recognised. In America, attention has for some time been turned to the problems of clothes for the handicapped. In this country the DLF has done some valuable work. It has had a Clothing Advisory Panel and projects on clothing problems since 1963. A survey of the situation has been published together with handbooks giving advice on different aspects of the problem (see p. 27). The Foundation has a Clothing Adviser and offers information on clothing in the form of demonstration collections, lecture/demonstrations, static exhibitions and modelled shows with commentaries. There are also notes on clothing problems which are updated regularly.

Despite more flexible attitudes to clothes and unisex fashions, most disabled women are more concerned about clothes than their male counterparts. The media, especially womens' magazines, stress the importance of appearance and clothes for women. Femininity is reflected in the way women dress. Most disabled women do not want to appear different from others in their social group. Yet women's clothes do present special difficulties for the disabled since they tend to be more complicated and difficult to put on, especially items like bras and tights. Difficulties with buttons and zips restrict the range of garments they can buy. With a few exceptions, special clothing for handicapped women does not exist in this country. Some specialised garments are produced by the hospital clothing manufacturers but few are obtainable through retail or mail order services. In any case many of these lack appeal, or look institutional and unfashionable. Many women reject the idea of specially designed garments because they feel that they draw attention to their handicap.

In many cases ordinary clothes can be used, or adapted, if a few simple rules are observed, which take into consideration the particular disability. For example, loose clothes with few fasteners, or easy to grasp toggle and frog fastening may be easier for those who have a limited range of movement or weak or deformed hands. Magnetic buttons are available in the USA but they are rather heavy and expensive to buy. Their use is still experimental but they may prove to be of value in the future. For those who have a hemiplegia or have had a head injury and perhaps have the use of only one hand, or become giddy when stooping, the simplest possible methods of dressing are advisable. Front fastening brassieres or the Kempner Fastener (from the DLF) are particularly useful. The latter, which is a strong hook and bar fastener is particularly useful for those who only have the use of one hand. Elastic shoe laces are also valuable since they remove the need to tie laced shoes each time they are put on. Shoulder strap retainers and lingerie clasps hold garment straps together on the shoulders and are also useful. Velcro, the touch and close fastener consists of two nylon strips, one a mass of tiny hooks and the other tiny loops. When put together the hooks grip the loops to give a secure closure, but the two strips can easily be separated by pulling them apart. For example any button-through garment can be adapted to Velcro fastening and still remain normal in appearance when the button holes are sewn up and the buttons sewn on top of them. A brassiere can be adapted to front fastening using Velcro. Velcro comes in a variety of colours and in widths of ¾ – 2 inches. It is extremely versatile and can be used as a straightforward fastener, in strips or dabs, as an alternative to buttons, zips and other fastenings. 'Dabs' of Velcro are far easier to open and close as they do not require such precise positioning or long range movement as a continuous strip of material. (Further information can be obtained from The Clothing Adviser at the DLF).

In general it is better to wear detail on the bodice, in particular on the neck and shoulder, rather than the skirt, as this draws attention away from calipers, surgical shoes etc. Trousers are often favoured by wheelchair users for warmth and to disguise calipers or deformed legs but they are not so convenient for toiletting purposes. Two-piece garments are generally more comfortable and convenient than one piece dresses. Wrap-round skirts which can be worn with the openings at the back or the front are useful and easy to put on, especially if Velcro is used at the waistline. They also have advantages when transferring from wheelchair to lavatory, if the opening is worn at the back. A button-through dress is practical for those who prefer a one-piece garment, but find it difficult to put a dress on over the head or to do up back fastenings. An adjustable waistline on skirts, trousers and dresses from maternity departments are helpful to wheelchair users who, as a result of prolonged sitting, have suffered a figure change. Tucked-in blouses should be long and made in stretchy materials which permit the wide range of shoulder and arm movement required for self-propelling and transferring from a wheelchair. A yoke or fullness over the shoulders can be useful but the former should be narrow since the seam restricts movement if it is lower down the back. Too much fullness at the cuffs, buttons and other fastenings tend to catch in the wheels of the chair and can be dangerous. Cuff protectors can be helpful in wet weather. A waterproof leg and lap cover can be supplied by the Department of Health and Social Security as an accessory for most wheelchairs designed for outdoor use. A cover which protects chair and occupant, the 'Wheelymac', can be obtained from Simplantex Ltd., Willowfield Road, Eastbourne, Sussex, BN22 8AR. Short coats, car coats and anoraks are useful for outdoor wear.

Dressing and undressing time and effort can be reduced by careful selection of garments and their fastenings. Independence in personal activities is a great boost to morale and a desirable goal to strive for, but the cost of achieving such independence must be carefully considered. Although it is gratifying to know that one can be independent, dressing without help, where such help is available, may not be making the best use of one's limited physical resources, particularly someone going to work or a mother with a family.

One of the greatest difficulties for women is the inconvenience or the impossibility of shopping for clothes. Too often there is no room to manoeuvre wheelchairs. Fitting rooms are awkward to enter and do not accommodate a wheelchair. Multiple stores which have their merchandise displayed in easily accessible ground floor accommodation and allow the customer to take goods on approval with a money-back guarantee are the most satisfactory. Mail order services can be very useful. (lists can be obtained from the DLF). Their well illustrated catalogues ensure that a careful choice of clothes can be made at home in quiet surroundings. Unsuitable goods may be exchanged or returned, but this presents difficulties to those who live alone if their handicap prevents them from wrapping the parcel and returning it by post. Current fashions should be watched, as there are often useful trends, which can be used or adapted by disabled women.

USEFUL PUBLICATIONS

P. Macartney, *Clothes Sense for Handicapped Adults of All Ages*, DLF 1973. Gives details of useful items of specialised garments which are obtainable. There are also suggestions for simple adaptations which can be undertaken at home. Helpful chapter on aids to independence, including fastenings, dressing techniques and aids.
How to Adapt Existing Clothing for the Disabled, DLF 1971. Sewing notes with illustrations.
E.E. Rogers and B.M. Stevens, *Dressmaking for the Disabled: adapting paper patterns to individual physical disabilities*, Association of Occupational Therapists 1966.
M.D. England, *Footwear for Problem Feet*, DLF 1973. Contains a great deal of useful advice on general problems of foot health and comfort.
Margery Thornton, *Footwear: what to get and where to get it*, DLF, Second edition 1979.

The above publications are all available in addition to information leaflets at the Disabled Living Foundation (see p. 43). For any further advice, write to the Clothing Adviser at the DLF.

Clothing and Dressing for Adults. This is a separate section in 'Equipment for the Disabled' from *Equipment For The Disabled*, 2 Foredown Drive, Portslade, Sussex BN4 2BB.
Comfortable Clothes. Details of a wide selection of garments especially designed for disabled people. All the garments have a normal appearance but special fastenings enable people to dress or be dressed more easily. The 1974 edition is still available from The Shirley Institute, Didsbury, Manchester M20 8RX, but unfortunately there is no likelihood of a further edition in the foreseeable future.

For advice on mastectomy (breast removal) clothing problems and prosthesis (artificial breast) write to **Mastectomy Association**, 1 Colworth Road, Croydon, Surrey.

8 Women at home

Over eighty-four per cent of all disabled women in Great Britain live at home. Amelia Harris estimated that sixty-eight per cent of these do their own housework to a greater or lesser degree. Therefore any effective aids, appliances or adaptations in the home can make life easier for a large percentage of these women. Indeed almost all the women in the Harris sample did most of the cooking. Three-quarters did most of the housework and two-thirds most of the shopping. Purpose-built or adapted accommodation can give the handicapped woman considerable independence in the home. The careful selection of aids ranging from simple or ingenious improvisations to sophisticated Possum equipment can greatly extend the range of activities. Where these can be combined with practical help regularly given in the form of home helps, district nurses etc., a remarkable degree of independence can often be achieved. In practice public expenditure cuts have meant that many of the aids and services have been restricted. For example, in 1977 Fay Wright of the Disability Alliance found that twenty-two per cent of local authorities were planning to cut their home help service and twenty-five per cent to reduce their meals-on-wheels. Aids and adaptations to the home have also been affected despite the Government's recommendation of an annual rise of nine per cent expansion rate of these services.

The Chronically Sick and Disabled Persons' Act 1970 requires local authorities to give the disabled person 'assistance in arranging for the carrying out of any works of adaptation in his home or any additional facilities designed to secure his greater safety, comfort or convenience'. This includes help to obtain wireless, television, library or similar recreational facilities and a telephone plus any special equipment necessary to use the instrument. In fact local authorities vary considerably in their interpretation of the Act, and the supply of aids and services differ from one part of the country to another. It is essential to find out how your local system works and approach the doctor or social worker (look up your local authority Social Services department in the telephone book) so that an occupational therapist can make a home visit to assess what help is necessary. Broadly speaking aids for independence in daily living activities should be supplied by the local authority social services department, whilst aids to nursing should be supplied by the area health authority through the National Health Service (contact your hospital or your GP). However it is often difficult to decide whether an aid is for personal independence or nursing purposes. For example, bath aids or a commode can be either, depending on the situation.

In some areas the disabled person is expected to pay part or all of the cost, depending on income. Wheelchairs are available through the appliance centres of the Department of Health and Social Security and although the prescription form must be signed by a hospital consultant or a GP, assessment is usually carried out by an occupational therapist or a physiotherapist working for the local authority or the area health authority. It is difficult to get financial help for some aids. Most social service departments will not pay for a washing machine even if it is essential for the disabled housewife to cope with the family wash, or a refrigerator for someone who can only go shopping, or, more likely, be taken shopping, once a week. Social workers may know of local charities which may be able to help with this sort of equipment.

For the disabled woman at home, planning and in particular the design of the kitchen and its equipment is vitally important. In fact well planned kitchens in most homes are the exception rather than the rule. Yet as Howie has pointed out, the handicap and hazard of badly planned and ill-equipped kitchens segregates the disabled housewife even more and exaggerates her difficulties, making it appear that special provision must always be made. Planning is improving and disabled women benefit particularly. A basic priority is the layout and design of the kitchen to minimise the problems of balancing, moving, stretching, stooping and carrying. A compact arrangement of work centres minimises lifting and moving. Cooker and sink should be sited together as the most frequent journeys are made between these two. Where the disabled woman is not wheelchair bound, a stool high enough to perch on or to take the weight off the feet is useful. Some women find a small stool or chair on wheels useful, as this allows them to sit to work and to move freely round the kitchen pushing with their feet.

Appropriate storage space needs to be near each work centre, but also mobile storage which can be moved to the place of need. Adjustable, shallow shelves, shelves which swing or pull out easily, shelving on the inside of cupboard doors, storage racks on wheels all have advantages. Trolleys are particularly useful. Split level cookers and micro-wave ovens are an advantage. (There has been discussion of cancer risk on these last). Adjustability of height cuts down the risk of burns. No cooker should have controls behind the pans, and eye-level grills are difficult for those who cannot reach or hold. A working surface is always needed near and at the same height as the boiling rings. Controls of light, meter, cooker, electric kettle and heaters must all be within easy reach. Refrigerators are a necessity but the small floor-based model may require a stand. Some Water Boards, including the Metropolitan, are willing to undertake modifications on the type and position of taps. Both British Gas and the Electricity Council offer special services for handicapped people. For example, every British Gas region employs Home Service Advisers who will visit the handicapped at home to advise on the use of gas appliances, including the free gas safety check which is available to disabled and elderly people who live alone, and includes minor repairs. All new cookers have automatic spark ignition, burners need no matches and pilot lights are becoming out-dated. On some new cookers, should the burner be accidentally extinguished, it will re-ignite at once. Various gas aids are detailed in a leaflet, *How Gas Makes Life Easier for Disabled People.* For women with hand disabilities there are special control adaptors which can be fitted to some cookers and fires. Pre-payment meters can be repositioned in a more convenient place, or special extension handles can be fitted or the meter changed from coin operation to a credit meter. The Electricity Council issue a useful little booklet called *Electric Aids for Disabled People* which covers a wide range of personal and domestic appliances.

Unfortunately many of the appliances to make living at home easier are expensive labour-saving devices or adaptations which require professional fitters. So, as Amelia Harris suggests, it is probably financial help that is most needed by those who wish to be independent and do their own housework. On the other hand she does report home-made adaptations or a different use of everyday objects. One woman had covered two bricks with adhesive plastic so that they would grip a bowl. Another used fire-tongs to get cakes out of the oven. A plumber's plastic plunger with five or six holes cut at regular intervals half an inch above the rim and then pushed up and down will give a gentle but thorough washing of 'smalls'. Or if gripping the handle of a knife or fork is a problem, it can be inserted into a bicycle handlebar grip which is cheap and easily obtained. Social service departments can often provide teapots and kettle tippers. The Red Cross publishes a book of aids which includes a pattern for a tipper. Rentoul make a good tipper from plastic covered wire which can be lifted from the back, pushed from the front, or both. (From Rentoul Workshops, Royal Cornwall Hospital, Infirmary Hill, Truro, Cornwall). A wooden one is quite easy to construct. There are now scissors available for the left-handed in the shops or small, snipping, spring-loaded scissors are easy to use with either hand. It is worth making an enquiry to 'Anything Left-Handed Ltd', at 65, Beak Street, London W1.

At the other end of the scale is the electronic remote control equipment, which is the biggest single advance towards enabling very severely disabled women have some control, and therefore independence, in their homes. The systems make use of any slight movement in head, hands or feet, or through a pneumatic switch operated by sucking and blowing to enable the disabled person to exercise control over a variety of electric appliances. The best known of these systems is 'Possum' (from the Latin, meaning 'I can' or 'I am able') which is available free of charge through the National Health Service to people approved by medical assessment. The basic unit usually consists of equipment to switch on/off devices such as lights, radio, television, door and intercom and also gives control over a loud-speaking telephone. The Post Office issue a leaflet (DLE 550) *Help for the Handicapped* which describes the latest developments. A new device is a pay-phone coin aid. It is designed to be operated by a handpull, or a lever pushed by the user's wheelchair and overcomes some of the problems of people who are mobility handicapped. The GPO are hoping that the popularity of press-button Keyphones, which are easier to operate than the conventional telephone is, will bring the cost down in the near future. The telephone, a vital link and means of communication for the handicapped woman at home, is a costly item, especially since cutbacks have meant that many local authorities have restricted the free provision of this service. A small consolation is that wall mounted telephones cost the same to instal as table models, can be placed at a convenient height for wheelchair users and are somewhat easier for dialling purposes.

Shopping seems to present more difficulties for many disabled women than any other activity. Yet it is often the activity which they miss most, and is a valuable form of social contact. Even if the disabled woman is able to get to the shops, wheelchair access into the shop is often difficult although this is improving. A common difficulty is having to stand in the shop. There are few shops with chairs for customers, but this situation could be easily remedied. The neighbourhood will determine what shops can be used. Supermarkets have advantages in that it is easy to see the goods, a trolley may give support, everything is under one roof and they have a large selection and are often cheaper. On the other hand many wheelchair users cannot reach and grasp goods on the shelves and find it difficult to pay and pack at the cash desk when queues form. Some women prefer the personal attention of the small local shop which takes into account personal difficulties and will often deliver goods. However, they often have less choice of goods and may be rather expensive. Bulk buying of foods, using refrigerators and freezers may be an answer for some women but it does require considerable financial outlay.

USEFUL PUBLICATIONS

Excellent literature is available. The DLF issues information sheets on subjects which include the following:— household equipment, beds, chairs, eating and drinking aids, personal toilet, personal aids etc.
Ed. S. Foott, *Kitchen Sense for Disabled or Elderly People*, DLF and Heinemann Medical Books 1975.
P.M. Howie, *Disabled Housewives in their Kitchens,* DLF 1967.
S. Foott, *Handicapped at Home,* Design Centre in association with DLF, 1977.
P. Nichols, *Living with a Handicap,* Priory Press Ltd., 49 Lansdowne Place, Hove, East Sussex 1973. Advice on aids.
RICA Comparative Test Reports. National Fund for Research into Crippling Diseases. Tests all kinds of household items from the point of view of the disabled user.
Aids to Independence, Royal Association of Disability and Rehabilitation (RADAR). Drawings for the making of aids and suggestions for overcoming handicaps.
Home-made Aids for Handicapped People, British Red Cross Society, revised edition 1974.
B. Ansell and S. Lawton, *Your Home and Your Rheumatism,* Arthritis and Rheumatism Council, second edition 1978.
Ian Earnshaw, *Disabled Housewives on Merseyside,* Disablement Income Group (DIG) 1973.

Education and employment

Education is a right for all. Society has a duty to ensure that disabled people are not prevented from enjoying this right. It may mean that measures of positive discrimination are employed so that the handicapped member is not disadvantaged in an educational system organised for the non-handicapped. Such measures apply both to disabled men and women, although perhaps females are encouraged less by families and schools to take advantage of further education opportunities. Too often those who have grown up with a handicap may find that their educational potential is under-assessed and it is assumed that they will remain at home. For the woman who becomes disabled later in life, further education and training may enable her to alter course to accommodate the handicap. A certain amount of practical help does exist.

For example, disabled students on mandatory award courses may claim a special allowance in addition to their normal grant. This allowance is in respect of additional expenditure caused by disability — for example special typewriters. It is very much up to local authorities to decide whether expenditure is necessarily incurred, but if in doubt go ahead and claim. Students on discretionary award courses can also apply for this allowance from their grant awarding body. In these cases an authority is not under an obligation to pay the allowance.

The Manpower Services Commission is responsible for all training and employment of disabled people. Financial support and free training is offered by the Manpower Services Commission (MSC) to people who want to undertake a course of training which will improve their employment prospects through the Training Opportunities Scheme (TOPS). Support under TOPS, which is open to both disabled and able-bodied people, is available in respect of a range of existing courses at Colleges of Further Education and courses especially set up by the Training Services Division of MSC. Training is also available at Skillcentres. Sometimes the eligibility conditions under TOPS are relaxed for handicapped people so that, for example, a disabled person can be accepted for training even though under nineteen years of age, and may be given a second course in less than five years. Disabled people also have special training opportunities under Other Training Arrangements (OTA) and the Professional Training Scheme (PTS). These may include training of longer than twelve months and training on an individual basis with an employer who is prepared to employ the trainee afterwards. A disabled person may be accepted for part-time training or for training by means of a correspondence course, including those of the Open University (see p.43). PTS provides assistance to disabled people who wish to train for a professional career, possibly involving a first degree, but who cannot obtain a normal educational grant. Graduates may be eligible for postgraduate courses but must be over twenty-seven years old. All courses taken under the TOPS scheme are free and trainees also receive a weekly tax-free allowance and other benefits such as travelling expenses, lunch, free credit of National Insurance contributions and an accommodation allowance for those who have to stay away from home.

Supplementary benefits legislation is rather more generous in its treatment of disabled students than of the able-bodied taking educational courses. For example, disabled students, whose prospects of employment are such that they would be unlikely to obtain a job if they were not in further education, can claim supplementary benefit during term-time if they have been refused a grant by their local authority. However, it is always better to apply for an education grant as these are more generous and the DHSS is unlikely to pay for tuition fees, books etc. Disabled students applying for supplementary benefit in term-time will be required to produce medical certificates at regular intervals. There are also several exceptional circumstances additions to supplementary benefits to which disabled students may be entitled, for example extra heating costs, special diets and high laundry bills.

For disabled people who need to be trained under residential conditions, MSC provides a variety of vocational courses in four residential colleges. They are intended to prepare disabled people for open employment in industry or commerce. Applications for any of the MSC courses should be made to the Disablement Resettlement Officer (DRO) who will be found in the local Job Centre or Employment Office. Useful leaflets can also be obtained. They are *Training for a Better Job with TOPS* (TSA L90), *Training Opportunities For Disabled People* (TSA L15), *Training Opportunities for Young Disabled People* (TSA L84) and *Residential Training for Disabled People* (TSA L65).

The National Star Centre for Disabled Youth is a unique institution, a specialised College of Further Education, recognised by the Department of Education and Science, offering courses to students with a wide range of physical handicap. The centre aims to provide courses varying in level from general remedial work to University studies. It is a recognised examinations centre for the Associated Examining Boards 'O' and 'A' levels and the Royal Society of Arts Examinations. The College, at Ullenwood Manor, near Cheltenham, has almost 100 students, from 16-35 years old, 60 per cent of them in wheelchairs. The current ratio of female to male students is 1 : 1.

The National Bureau for Handicapped Students (Thomas Coram Foundation, 40 Brunswick Square, London WC1, Telephone 01-278 3127) was formed in 1975 to help and advise disabled students, to collect information to formulate policy matters and to publicise the educational needs of handicapped people. The Bureau, which publishes a termly newsletter *Educare,* aims to establish links with all further educational establishments in the United Kingdom. Already over 450 such institutions have become members of the Bureau and many are actively involved in its work. Their work is likely to become even more important because of the increasing emphasis on mature students, which has important implications for disabled students.

As with education, in theory women have equal opportunity with men in employment. In practice women are often discriminated against in the labour market. This is even more so in the case of disabled women, where it may be assumed that they are content to stay at home. Disabled women are also less likely to be registered as disabled than men. It is advisable for any woman who is disabled, or who becomes disabled and wants to explore work possibilities, to see her Disablement Resettlement Officer (DRO) at the Job Centre or Employment office as quickly as possible. There are over 500 DROs all over the country to advise disabled people about employment and to help them find it. This service has been much criticised, and certainly it is often ineffective, but it is the link with all the other facilities provided by the Manpower Services Commission. The MSC has the responsibility for training and employment services for disabled people. These services include the Job Introduction Scheme which gives employers a weekly grant for a trial period, normally six weeks, so that they can employ a disabled person who needs to prove ability. Studies have shown that four out of every five helped this way continued to hold their jobs after the trial period. Another scheme makes available grants for modifications to premises and equipment when this is essential for the recruitment or retention of disabled employees. Take-up of these schemes by employers is very low, but imaginative and well-publicised use could be of enormous benefit to disabled women.

The individual disabled person can also receive direct assistance from MSC, for example assistance with travel to work. Following the changes in mobility policy, which included the introduction of a weekly cash allowance, the phasing out of the invalid vehicle and the setting up of 'Motability' (an organisation to help people convert their cash into cars) the MSC has revised its fares-to-work scheme. Financial assistance, usually a contribution of 75 per cent towards taxi costs, is given to people who can neither drive nor be driven, nor use public transport to get to work. The number of aids issued to disabled people in open employment is increasing every year. They include special desks and chairs, adapted typewriters, dictation machines and tape recorders. Firms such as Gestetner are developing ways in which their machinery can be adapted to accommodate people with a wide range of disabilities. The British Computer Society has a Specialist Group for the Disabled to inform disabled people of employment opportunities. Among their projects Aptitude Testing and Training for disabled people.

There is a great need for information about individual solutions to employment problems to be made widely available for the benefit of others with similar problems. For the disabled professional there is The Association of Disabled Professionals (ADP). They stress that no one is too disabled to work and that there are few professions which cannot be followed by disabled people, no matter how severely disabled they may be.

Many disabled women seek outlets to counterbalance their physical limitations. Their mental and physical frustrations channel themselves into the desire to use to the full the abilities they do have. They desperately need the stimulus, satisfaction and independence which comes from being able to work, preferably outside the home, but if this is impossible, then at home. Many people think of working at home as exploitation and being limited to factory outwork or envelope addressing. In fact the scope can be surprisingly wide, as indicated by Joanna Johnson in her excellent *Working At Home*, now unfortunately out of print. Joanna, who is disabled, describes herself as a 'home worker extraordinary' and has done many different types of housebound employment, including an academic typing service and freelance journalism. Some professions do lend themselves more easily to home work. For example a teacher can offer private coaching or examination marking. With the relevant qualifications, freelance editing, indexing, technical writing, translating, statistical analysis of data can be undertaken. Housebound computer programmers can have direct telephone access to computers installed by the GPO.

Home Opportunities for Professional Employment (HOPE) is a small organisation, virtually run by one person who collects information on the possibilities of working at home for people who have had to give up their professional careers. Information can be obtained from Ronald Gerver, the Honorary Secretary, at 96 Greencroft Gardens, London NW6. Many commercial firms offer home work which may be suitable for disabled women. It is wise to investigate thoroughly any firm offering home work. Many exploit their workers financially. Advice can be obtained from The Homeworkers Association, 9 Poland Street, London W1V 3DG.

Whatever the level of ability and qualifications the disabled woman, eager and able to work, will have to be imaginative and persistent in her pursuit of the opportunities which do exist both through the services of MSC and the voluntary organisations. For it is a fact of life, however regrettable, that in the search for work the disabled woman is more discriminated against than the disabled man. However, ironically, because of the non-manual and traditional nature of what is regarded as women's spheres of activity it is often easier for women to adapt than men.

USEFUL PUBLICATIONS

Educational Charities NUS.
Financial Assistance for Disabled Students NUS & The National Bureau for Handicapped Students 1978.
D. Child and G. Markall, *The Disabled Student,* NUS & Action Research for the Crippled Child 1976.
Access to University and Polytechnic Buildings: a handbook for disabled students, RADAR 1977.
An Educational Policy for Handicapped People, National Bureau for Handicapped Students 1977.
Joanna Johnson, *Working at Home*, A Penguin handbook 1971. Now out of print but may be obtainable at libraries.
Henry Mara and Penny Thrift, *Get Yourself Going,* 1977. An Action Handbook for the Handicapped Office Worker. Useful information for disabled people who want to earn a living in an office or run a business at home. Available from RADAR.
Maxwell Crooks, *Special Typewriter Keyboard Charts and Instructions for Handicapped Typists,* National Fund for Research into Crippling Diseases
Nina Richardson, *Type With One Hand,* Cincinnati South Western Publishing Company 1959. Available from American Book Service, Amersham, Bucks.
Bernadette Fallon, *Able to Work,* Spinal Injuries Association 1979

10 Benefits

It is well known and documented that the disabled find it much more difficult to manage financially than the able bodied because of the extra costs of disability. Yet the average disabled person has a lower income than the average able bodied person and is less likely to be employed. This is still the situation, despite new benefits introduced by successive governments in recent years. Indeed the system which has now become so complex and full of anomalies, was the subject of a recent book, *Whose Benefit* (see p. 41). Despite the new benefits, it is true to say that the present system is based on the *cause* of disablement rather than its *effect,* so that contribution record, age, sex, place of injury are more important than degree of incapacity and need. So different people, who are equally disabled, are entitled to a wide range of income benefit, or even none at all. Women are traditionally disadvantaged in our social security system. Disabled women, particularly if they are married, suffer most of all.

Some benefits however, are universal.

Attendance Allowance is payable to both men and women who require regular help in fulfilling their physical needs. It is paid tax free, at a higher rate for day *and* night care, at a lower rate for day *or* night care. Only the most severely disabled will qualify.

Invalid Care Allowance is payable to a husband or other relative who cannot go to work because they are looking after, full-time, a person receiving an Attendance Allowance.

Similarly, the **Mobility Allowance** is a universal benefit for the disabled under pension age, intended to help with the costs of transport for those who are unable to walk.

Supplementary benefit is a non-contributory means-tested benefit payable to those whose income falls below the scale rate determined annually by parliament. It does not apply to married women or women who are cohabiting, who will get nothing.
Exceptional circumstances additions (ECAs) may be added to the weekly payment in respect of heating, laundry, diet and other recurring costs. Occasional **Exceptional Needs Payments** (ENPs) may be granted for essentials such as clothing and are available to those with very little capital even if they do not receive supplementary benefit. Disabled people often receive other benefits, which are also available to the able-bodied, such as unemployment benefit, family income supplement, etc., providing they fulfil the conditions.

Details of how to claim these benefits and claim forms can be obtained from any social security office.

However, the principle means of income support for the disabled is **Invalidity Benefit,** payable to those who have paid National Insurance stamps in the past and have been receiving sickness benefit for 28 weeks. As a contributory benefit, and as many women do not pay contributions, it inevitably works against women. The **Non-contributory Invalidity Pension** (NCIP) began in 1975. It was designed to cover an estimated 220,000 men and single women of working age who had become sick or disabled before they had been able to accumulate enough contributions to claim sickness and invalidity benefits, and were therefore in all probability relying on long-term supplementary benefit. The government made it clear that disabled married women were to be excluded, but a backbench revolt at the Committee stage of the Social Security Act 1975, which introduced the NCIP, forced the Government to extend the new legislation to cover married women. However, whereas men and single women have only to prove that they are incapable of paid employment, a married or cohabiting woman is required to satisfy the DHSS that she is also 'incapable of performing normal household duties'. Yet the National Insurance Advisory Committee, to whom the draft Housewives Non-contributory Invalidity Pension (HNCIP) regulations were submitted for approval, reported that 'the majority of the organisations from which we received representations expressed their opinion that the provisions in the Act which relate to the non-contributory invalidity pension unfairly discriminate against married women and they asked us to consider recommending that the Act should be amended so as to permit married women to claim benefit on equal terms with men and single women'.

The number of women concerned is considerable. The Government estimated that about 40,000 women would be eligible for HNCIP. By May 1978, 35,000 women were receiving it. There is no reliable estimate as to how many disabled women would be eligible if it were not for the household duties test, but it could be as high as 100,000. By June 1978, 9,400 women incapable of paid work, that is about 15 per cent of those who claimed, had been refused HNCIP because of the test.

To date the DHSS has been unable to give a workable definition of what is meant by incapacity to perform 'normal household duties'. The National Insurance Commissioner stated that it was 'a subjective test, in that it is the claimants' own incapacity for normal household duties which is to be considered, judged, however, by reference to the objective standard of the duties which a capable housewife would perform were she in the claimants' situation, in that particular household and that environment'. The claim form itself is complicated, with twenty-five sections to complete, some of which can easily be misinterpreted. In a recent case a local tribunal awarded a disabled woman HNCIP, but the DHSS appealed on the grounds that as she could do many light household tasks, she could not qualify. However, the Tribunal held that the regulations were concerned not with what a woman is able to do, but what she is unable to do. Their view of the test was whether a woman 'is effectively prevented from running her household in the manner to be expected of a housewife in her circumstances and to maintain it to the standard appropriate to such circumstances'.

At present the situation is that if a woman is incapable of doing by herself, even with the use of aids and appliances, almost all of the jobs which normally fall to a housewife, or if she can do some of these jobs but only with great difficulty, slowness and pain, she can apply. In view of the DHSS policy it is advisable to emphasise the jobs that cannot be done unaided, rather than those which can. The claim has to be supported by a medical report and then passed to the insurance officer at the DHSS for a decision. If a claim is refused, an appeal can be made to a local appeal tribunal and the procedure will be explained in a letter from the insurance officer. It is always worthwhile making an appeal, since over 52 per cent are successful. Yet many women do not appeal when they are turned down, although they seem to have a good case. Different tribunals reach opposite decisions in virtually identical cases, and women who are not represented at the hearing appear to have little chance of succeeding. A final appeal can be made to the National Insurance Commissioner.

Obviously HNCIP is unacceptable in its present form, based as it is on the outdated assumptions about the position of married women as their husband's dependants. In the last twenty-five years, the proportion of married women in the labour market has more than doubled. It is expected to be 55 per cent by 1986. In a survey of a group of disabled married women (see p. 41), almost all the 200 women had been assessed as being unable to go out to work but had been refused HNCIP. In other words, they were being discriminated against because they happened to be married or living with a man as his wife. Any married woman who is incapable of taking paid work should be entitled to NCIP in the same way as any other disabled person. Secondly, HNCIP is unacceptable because it penalises disabled women who try to help themselves and retain their physical independence in the home. It encourages women with progressive diseases to give up trying and discourages others from trying to rehabilitate themselves.

Eda Topliss has shown that families with a disabled housewife appear to suffer financially almost as much as those where the breadwinner is disabled. It was not, in most cases, because the husband had given up work to care for the wife but rather that they were unable to do overtime or their domestic burdens reduced their promotion opportunities. Most importantly, the disabled wives were unlikely to be employed so they lacked the second income that is now so common in marriage. Yet the unavoidable extra expenses of disablement for this group are obvious — for example, washing, mending and making do are often difficult or impossible. Then there is the cost of paying others to collect, escort or care for children, or the extra expense of not being able to shop around, and so on. One of the most disturbing facts to emerge from Mavis Hyman's study is that 20 to 50 per cent of total household income may be spent on extra expenses due to the disability of one member.

Until the legislation is altered, all women who think they may qualify for HNCIP should apply, concentrating, on the form, on those tasks they cannot do, and if they are rejected, making an appeal. Advice can be sought from 'Equal Rights for Disabled Women Campaign' at 5 Netherhall Gardens, London NW3. Representing a wide variety of groups, they are campaigning for the abolition of the 'household duties' test and for married women to be paid NCIP on the same basis as all other disabled people. It is not only HNCIP which needs to be amended. A simplification of the whole complex system of disability benefits is long overdue. The Disablement Income Group (DIG) a national voluntary organisation campaigning to improve the situation of all disabled people was itself founded in 1965 by two disabled housewives who discovered on becoming disabled that no assistance was available to them. The most urgent need is for a tax free disablement allowance based on the sole criterion of incapacity, which provides for the extra costs of disabled living and the changing role of women in our society.

USEFUL PUBLICATIONS

Help for Handicapped People is a booklet (free) on benefits and services available from any office of the DHSS.
Jean Simkins and Vincent Tickner, *Whose Benefit*, DIG and Economist Intelligence Unit Ltd 1978.
Disability Rights Handbook, The Disability Alliance 1979 (published annually)
ABC of Services and Information for Disabled People, Disablement Income Group 1978 (published annually)
Irene Loach and Ruth Lister, *Second Class Disabled*, Equal Rights for Disabled Women Campaign 1978.
Irene Loach, *Disabled Married Women*, The Disability Alliance 1977
Mavis Hyman, *The Extra Costs of Disabled Living*, DIG and the National Fund for Research into Crippling Diseases 1977.

11 Where to get advice and help

Action For The Disabled, 26 Barker Walk, Mt Ephraim Road, London SW16 (01-677 1276)
Arthritis And Rheumatism Council, 8-10 Charing Cross Road, London WC2H 0HN (01-240 0871)
Association For Spina Bifida And Hydrocephalus, Tavistock House North, Tavistock Square, London WC1 (01-388 1382)
Association For Independent Disabled Self-Sufficiency, 7 Alfred Street, Bath BA1 2QU, Avon. An organisation to bring support, , both financial and non-material, to the lives of all categories of disabled people, Bath (0225) 25197.
Association Of Disabled Professionals, Tavistock House South, Tavistock Square, London WC1H 9LB (01-387 4037)
British Association Of Myasthenics, 49 Main Street, Dunshalt, Cupar, Fife, Scotland (Auchtermuchty 529)
British Computer Society, (Specialist Group for the Disabled), 29 Portland Place, London W1 4HU (01-637 0471)
British Polio Fellowship, Bell Close, West End Road, Ruislip, Middlesex (71-75515)
British Red Cross Society, 9 Grosvenor Crescent, London SW1X 7EJ (01-235 5454)
British Rheumatism And Arthritis Association, 6 Grosvenor Crescent, London SW1X 7ER (01-235 0902)
Chest, Heart And Stroke Association, Tavistock House North, Tavistock Square, London WC1H 9JE (01-387 3012)
Committee On Sexual Problems Of The Disabled, (SPOD), 49 Victoria Street, London SW1 (01-222 6067)
Consumers Association, 14 Buckingham Street, London WC2 (01-930 9921)
Department of Health & Social Security, (DHSS), Alexander Fleming House, Elephant & Castle, London SE1 (01-407 5522)
Disabled Drivers' Association, Ashwellthorpe Hall, Ashwellthorpe, Norwich, Norfolk NR16 1EX (0508-41449)
Disabled Drivers' Motor Club, 39 Templewood, London W13 8DU (01-998 1226)
Disablement Income Group, (DIG), Attlee House, Toynbee Hall, 28 Commercial Street, London E1 6R (01-247 2128 and 247 6877)
Disability Alliance, 5 Netherhall Gardens, London NW3 5RN (01-794 1536)

Disabled Living Foundation, (DLF), 346 Kensington High Street, London W14 (01-602 2491) The Disabled Living Foundation (DLF) is a charitable trust whose terms of reference include all disabilities. The DLF works in those aspects of ordinary life which present specific problems and difficulties to disabled people of all ages and disabilities. Research projects, an information service and a comprehensive aids centre are some of the many activities of the foundation.
Family Planning Association, (FPA), 27-35 Mortimer Street, London W1N.7RJ (01-636 7866)
Gemma, BM Box 5700, London WC1V 6XX
Gaycare, 2a Thirlmere Road, Streatham, London SW16
Homeworkers' Association, 9 Poland Street, London W1V 3OG (01-437 1780)
International Cerebral Palsy Society, 5a Netherhall Gardens, London NW3 5RN (01-794 9761)
Masectomy Association, 1 Colworth Road, Croydon, Surrey CR0 7AD (01-654 8643)
Multiple Sclerosis Society Of Great Britain And Northern Ireland, 4 Tachbrook Street, London SW1V 1SJ (01-834 8231)
Muscular Dystrophy Group Of Great Britain, Natrass House, 35 Macaulay Road, London SW4 0QP (01-720 8055)
National Bureau For Handicapped Students, Thomas Coram Foundation, 40 Brunswick Square, London WC1N 1AZ (01-278 3127)
National Council For The Single Woman And Her Dependents. 29 Chilworth Mews, London W2 3RG. Organisation for women caring for elderly parents. (01-262 1451)
National Fund For Research Into Crippling Diseases, Vincent House, 1 Springfield Road, Horsham, West Sussex, RH12 2PN (0403-64101)
National Star Centre For Disabled Youth, Ullenwood Manor, Cheltenham, GLOS. (Cheltenham 27631)
National Union Of Students, (NUS), 302 Pentonville Road, London N1 9LD (01-278 3291)
Open University, Milton Keynes, MK7 6AB (Milton Keynes 74066)
Possum Users' Association, Copper Beech, Parry's Close, Stoke Bishop, Bristol BS9 1AW (0272-683596)
Royal Association For Disability And Rehabilitation, (RADAR), 25 Mortimer Street, London W1N 8AB (01-637 5400)
Scottish Committee For The Welfare Of The Disabled, 19 Claremont Crescent, Edinburgh EH7 4QD (031-556 3882)
Scottish Council For Spastics, 22 Corstorphine Road, Edinburgh EH12 6HP (031-337 2809)
Scottish Information Service For The Disabled, 18 Claremont Crescent, Edinburgh EH7 4QD (031-556 3882)

Scottish Paraplegic Association, 3 Cargill Terrace, Edinburgh EH5 3ND (031-552 8459)
Scottish Spina Bifida Association, 190 Queensferry Road, Edinburgh (031-332 0743)
Spastics Society, 12 Park Crescent, London W1N 4EQ (01-636 5020)
Spinal Injuries Association, 126 Albert Street, London NW1 7NF (01-267 6111)
Wales Council For The Disabled, Llys Ifor, Crescent Road, Caerphilly, Mid-Glamorgan, CF8 1XL (0222-869224)

FURTHER READING

M. Blaxter, *The Meaning of Disability, a sociological study of impairment*, Heinemann 1976.
D. Boswell and J. Wingrove eds, *The Handicapped Person in the Community*, Open University Set Book 1974.
A. Darnbrough and D. Kinrade, eds, *Directory for the Disabled*, Published in association with The Multiple Sclerosis Society, Woodhead-Faulkner 1977. A handbook of information and opportunities for the disabled.
B. Fallon, *So You're Paralysed*, Spinal Injuries Association 1975.
C. Faulder, *Talking to your Doctor*, Virago 1978.
E. Goffman, *Stigma: notes on the management of spoiled identity*, Pelican 1968.
A. Harris et al, *Handicapped and Impaired in Great Britain*, OPCS, HMSO 1971.
P. Jay, *Coping With Disablement*, Consumers Association 1974.
D. Lees and S. Shaw, eds, *Impairment, Disability and Handicap: a multidisciplinary view*, Heinemann 1974.
S. Mattingly ed, *Rehabilitation Today*, Update Books 1977.
M.A. Rogers, *Paraplegia: a handbook of practical care and advice*, Faber 1978.
S. Sainsbury, *Registered As Disabled*, Bell 1970.
E. Topliss, *Provision For the Disabled*, Blackwell 1975.